Nutritional Care of Older People

Also available from M&K Publishing

All books can be ordered online at: www.mkupdate.co.uk

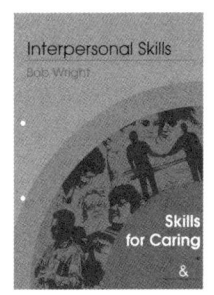

Interpersonal Skills Workbook
Bob Wright, RN, RMN, MSc (Leeds)
ISBN: 978-1-905539-37-6
Experienced professionals and novice care workers alike need to communicate meaningfully with their clients. To do so successfully you need to understand the skills required and how to practise them.

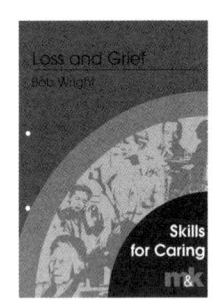

Loss & Grief Workbook
Bob Wright, SRN, RMN, MSc (Leeds)
ISBN: 978-1-905539-43-7
The feelings and thoughts connected with loss, grief, dying and death have always concerned people. The author Bob is a specialist in crisis intervention. He has developed his experience in counselling and as a workshop facilitator over a number of years. This updated self-directed study workbook will appeal to everyone with a health and social care interest.

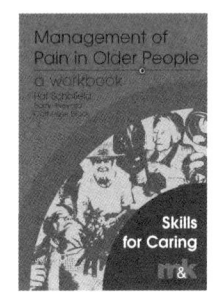

Management of Pain in Older People Workbook
ISBN: 978-1-905539-22-2
Dr Pat Schofield, Centre for Advanced Studies in Nursing, University of Aberdeen This workbook is not designed to make you an expert in pain management, but to increase your awareness of the complexity of the pain experience when working with older adults and to help you to understand the need for a creative and innovative approach to dealing with the person in your care who may be in pain.

Issues in Heart Failure Nursing
ISBN: 978-1-905539-00-0

The Management of COPD in Primary and Secondary Care
ISBN: 978-1-905539-28-4

The Clinician's Guide to Chronic Disease Management for Long-term Conditions
A cognitive-behavioural approach
ISBN: 978-1-905539-15-4

Routine Blood Results Explained
ISBN: 978-1-905539-38-3

Nurse Facilitated Hospital Discharge
ISBN: 978-1-905539-12-3

Improving Patient Outcomes
ISBN: 978-1-905539-06-2

Visit the M&K website for a full listing of titles in print and forthcoming books.

Forthcoming titles include:

Primary Care Case Studies for Nurse Practitioners
ISBN: 978-1-905539-23-9

Legal Principles and Clinical Practice
ISBN: 978-1-905539-32-1

Microbiology and Infection Investigations & Results
ISBN: 978-1-905539-36-9

Nutritional Care of Older People
a workbook

Amanda Taylor
BSc Hons PGDip RD

Nutritional Care of Older People Workbook
Amanda Taylor
ISBN: 978-1-905539-05-5
First published 2008

All rights reserved. No part of this publication may be reproduced, stored in a retrieval system, or transmitted in any form or by any means, electronic, mechanical, photocopying, recording or otherwise, without either the prior permission of the publishers or a licence permitting restricted copying in the United Kingdom issued by the Copyright Licensing Agency, 90 Tottenham Court Road, London, W1T 4LP. Permissions may be sought directly from M&K Publishing, phone: 01768 773030, fax: 01768 781099 or email: publishing@mkupdate.co.uk

Any person who does any unauthorised act in relation to this publication may be liable to criminal prosecution and civil claims for damages.

British Library Catalogue in Publication Data
A catalogue record for this book is available from the British Library

Notice
Clinical practice and medical knowledge constantly evolve. Standard safety precautions must be followed, but, as knowledge is broadened by research, changes in practice, treatment and drug therapy may become necessary or appropriate. Readers must check the most current product information provided by the manufacturer of each drug to be administered and verify the dosages and correct administration, as well as contraindications. It is the responsibility of the practitioner, utilising the experience and knowledge of the patient, to determine dosages and the best treatment for each individual patient. Any brands mentioned in this book are as examples only and are not endorsed by the Publisher. Neither the publisher nor the author assume any liability for any injury and/or damage to persons or property arising from this publication.

The Publisher
To contact M&K Publishing write to:
M&K Update Ltd · The Old Bakery · St. John's Street
Keswick · Cumbria CA12 5AS
Tel: 01768 773030 · Fax: 01768 781099
publishing@mkupdate.co.uk
www.mkupdate.co.uk

Designed & typeset by Mary Blood

Contents

List of figures and tables **vii**

About the author **viii**

Introduction **ix**

1 What is a healthy diet? **1**

2 Malnutrition and monitoring people who may be at risk of malnutrition **6**

3 Food fortification and nutritional supplements **17**

4 Special dietary needs **22**

5 Ethnicity, religion and culture **33**

6 Relevant policy guidelines and standards **35**

Appendix 1 **41**
Diet History Chart

Appendix 2 **43**
Food Record Chart

Appendix 3 **45**
Weight Chart

Appendix 4 **47**
Checklist for Best Practice – social care

Appendix 5 **49**
Checklist for Best Practice – hospital wards

Further reading **51**

References **53**

Figures

1.1 The eatwell plate **1**

Tables

1.1 Food groups **2**

1.2 Portions of fruit and vegetables **3**

2.1 Effects of malnutrition **6**

2.2 Factors in malnutrition **7**

2.3 What are the warning signs that a patient may be at risk of malnutrition and what action might I take? **10**

4.1 Reading food labels **23**

5.1 Religious food restrictions **33**

5.2 Sources of nutrients for Vegan diet **34**

Charts

2.1 Example of a food record chart that is not filled in correctly **13**

2.2 Example of a food record chart that is filled in correctly **14**

ABOUT THE AUTHOR

Amanda Taylor is a registered dietitian. This workbook draws on her experience working with older people, both as a dietitian and as a healthcare assistant in domiciliary care, nursing homes and in the acute setting.

Introduction

The UK population is ageing. The percentage of people aged 65 and over increased from 13 to 16 per cent between mid-1971 and mid-2005. Within this age group even greater increases were seen for those aged 85 and over. The number of people aged 85 and over grew by 64,000 (6 per cent) in the year to 2005 to reach a record 1.2 million. Population ageing will continue during the first half of this century, since the proportion of the population aged 65 and over will increase as the large numbers of people born after the Second World War become older (ONS, 2006). Ageing is a natural process involving physiological and biochemical changes that affect the whole of the body. The rate of decline in the body's functions as a result of ageing varies from person to person. Good nutrition contributes to the health of elderly people and their ability to maintain their independence, mobility and overall quality of life for longer. Ultimately, these factors may also lessen the burden of health costs.

The public and the press are very interested in food, especially food in hospitals and other institutions. Nutrition issues and older people's experiences of food and drink in various care settings have been highlighted as areas that should be given more attention, as a result of various campaigns such as the Department of Health Dignity in Care survey of 2006 (Department of Health 2006), and the Report Hungry in Hospital? (Association of Community Health Councils of England and Wales, 1997). Several participants in the Dignity in Care online survey described occasions when they had witnessed vulnerable service users being left alone at meal times with no support or assistance to eat their meals. Respondents commented that carers did not seem to have time to spend with individuals at meal times or that they were unobservant and had failed to notice that a service user needed help. Meal times seemed to be a process to be got over with as quickly as possible rather than potentially a sociable opportunity. Some service users may be embarrassed to ask for help, therefore, survey respondents said that care staff should be more aware of what people's needs are at meal times. Many people said that they found it distressing to see a vulnerable adult not being able to eat their own meals and it was perceived as a sign of neglect in some institutions.

The food that is provided in hospitals and care homes can define the whole experience of the organisation for the patient (or service user). They may or may not be able to tell the difference between good or bad treatment, but can always tell if the food is good or bad. Food has a role quite apart from its primary function to provide the body with fuel and nutrients to stay alive. When we celebrate a happy occasion food usually features – birthday cake, wedding breakfast to name two examples. Workers look forward to lunch break, when they can experience a change of scenery or socially interact with different people for a while. Meal times in hospitals, care homes and residential homes can also mark a break in a long and uneventful day. They should be treated as such, and protected meal times are a way of ensuring that people are given enough time to enjoy their meals, and give staff enough time to assist those who require it. The environment and ambience of a ward can make a dramatic difference to how the food is perceived and the amounts eaten.

It is not only in hospitals and care homes that carers are concerned with the food and nutrition of older people. Care staff who look after clients in their own homes can make a significant contribution to their nutritional care. The carer may be the only person the client sees on a daily basis, and often the carer is a lone worker. One of the objectives of this workbook is to facilitate the lone worker to engage in communication with colleagues as well as service users and their families, to ensure that nutrition is regarded as an integral part of care. When a care worker is not working alone but as part of a team on a ward or in a care home, it may be unclear who is directly responsible for nutritional care. The answer is simple – you are! This book has been written to heighten awareness of nutrition as care and encourage readers to take ownership of ensuring that good practice is implemented on a day to day basis. You will find that completing the exercises will improve your understanding of what nutritional care means to your client group whether they are in hospital, residential care or in their own home.

A Brief Note About Consent

You will notice that there are reminders throughout the text, especially with regard to completing the exercises, to gain consent from the patient or family, and refer to your organisation's record keeping and documentation policies.

1 What is a Healthy Diet?

KEY POINTS

- By including a large variety of foods individuals will take in a wide variety of nutrients.
- Healthy elderly people should, when possible, follow the same healthy eating guidelines as the rest of the adult population.
- Special consideration should be given to calcium, vitamin D and vitamin C.

The body requires a variety of different foods every day, in order to take in all the nutrients required to help it to function efficiently. This may be termed a 'balanced diet'.

Fig 1.1
The eatwell plate

The eatwell plate

Use the eatwell plate to help you get the balance right. It shows how much of what you eat should come from each food group.

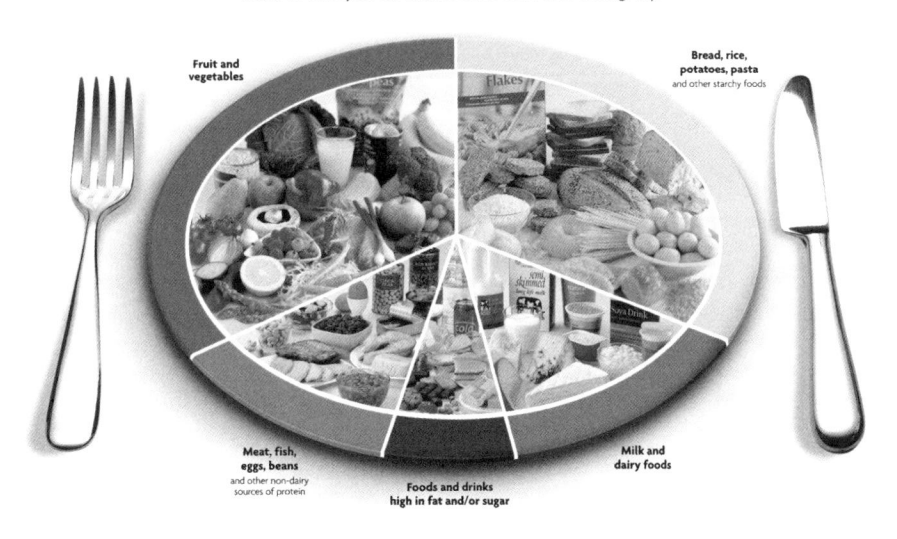

Source: Office of Public Sector Information. Used with permission (licence number V2007000553).

There are five main food groups, which are shown in Figure 1.1, and detailed in Table 1.1. By including a large variety of the foods listed in Table 1.1 individuals will take in a wide variety of nutrients.

A guide to the amount of food from each group that should be eaten is as follows:

- Plenty of fruit and vegetables – at least five portions per day.
- Plenty of bread, rice, potatoes, pasta and other starchy foods; wholegrain varieties should be chosen whenever possible.
- Milk and dairy foods should be eaten every day.
- Some meat, fish, eggs, beans and other non-dairy sources of protein should be eaten every day.

What is a healthy diet?

- Foods and drinks high in fat and/or sugar should be enjoyed occasionally.
- Fish – it is recommended that two portions per week should be eaten, one of which should be oily.

Table 1.1
Food groups

	Main Foods	**Nutrients Provided**
Bread, other cereals and potatoes	Whole grain varieties of bread and cereals are a healthier choice, as they contain complex carbohydrates which are released into the blood more slowly. Other cereals means foods such as breakfast cereals, pasta, rice, oats, noodles, maize, millet and cornmeal. Beans and pulses can be eaten as part of this group.	Carbohydrate (starch) Fibre Some calcium and iron B Vitamins
Fruit and vegetables	Fresh, frozen, dried and canned fruit. Fresh, frozen and canned vegetables. One glass of fruit juice per day also counts. Beans and pulses can be eaten as part of this group.	Vitamin C Carotenes Folate
Milk and dairy foods	Milk, cheese, yoghurt and fromage frais. This group does not include butter, eggs and cream.	Calcium Protein Vitamin B12 Vitamins A and D
Meat, fish and alternatives	Meat, poultry, fish, eggs, nuts, beans, pulses, soya and quorn. Meat includes bacon and meat products such as sausages, pies and burgers.	Iron Protein B Vitamins, especially B12 Zinc Magnesium
Foods containing fat and sugar	Margarine, butter, other spreading fats and low fat spreads, cooking oils, oil-based salad dressings, mayonnaise, cream, chocolate, crisps, pastries, cakes, puddings, ice cream, rich sauces, sweets, desserts, jam, biscuits and soft drinks.	Fat, including some essential fatty acids, but also some vitamins. Some products also contain salt or sugar.

By 2020 it is expected that 25% of the population in Europe will be aged over 60. It is recommended that healthy elderly people should, when possible, follow the same healthy eating guidelines as the rest of the adult population. However special consideration should be given to calcium, vitamin D and vitamin C.

Table 1.2
Portions of fruit and vegetables

Fruit and Vegetables	What is a portion?
Whole fresh fruit, e.g. apple, orange, pear	1 fruit
Large fruit	1 slice melon/pineapple 1/2 grapefruit
Small fruit	12 grapes, 2 plums, 2 kiwi, 7 strawberries
Dried fruit	1 dessertspoon
Tinned fruit in juice/stewed fruit, e.g. apple, rhubarb	3 large tablespoons
Fruit juice	1 small glass or carton
Vegetables, e.g. cauliflower, cabbage, broccoli, swede, peppers	2 large tablespoons
Salad	1 small bowl
Tomato	1 medium size

CALCIUM AND VITAMIN D

In people aged over 50, osteoporosis and the fractures that result from it are a major cause of illness and death. The Department of Health recommends that adults should take in 700mg of calcium per day in the form of milk and milk-based foods, fortified bread and breakfast cereals and vegetables. The body requires vitamin D in order to absorb calcium. Vitamin D is produced in the body by the action of sunlight on the skin. Older people are at risk of vitamin D deficiency, as the skin's ability to manufacture vitamin D from sunlight declines with age. Also, some older people tend not to go outdoors very often, and those who do may be covered or sheltered from the sun. Vitamin D can be obtained in the diet from oily fish (mackerel, kippers, salmon, pilchards) and it is recommended that these should be eaten twice a week.

VITAMIN C

Fruit and vegetables are the main source of vitamin C in the diet. It is recommended that they should make up about one-third of the daily diet. This can include fresh, frozen and tinned fruit and vegetables and pure fruit juice. Older people may be deterred from aiming for five portions of fruit and vegetables due to difficulty in peeling and cutting such foods. They may find it difficult to chew certain fruits, especially with the skin on. You can encourage elderly clients to eat more fruit and vegetables in the following ways:

What is a healthy diet?

- A piece of chopped (and peeled if appropriate) fruit can be offered as a snack.
- Clients can be encouraged to have a glass of pure fruit juice with one meal a day.
- Stewed fruit can be served with custard, yoghurt or ice cream for a dessert.
- Dried fruits can be added to porridge and cereals.

Vitamin C is an important nutrient for wound healing and it also improves the body's absorption of iron.

POINTS FOR REFLECTION

Do you think your patients/clients are managing to eat a well-balanced diet?

EXERCISE 1

Write in the space below what a balanced diet may consist of over the course of a day. Use the information from Figure 1.1 and Tables 1.1 and 1.2.

Breakfast

Lunch

Evening Meal

Snacks

What is a healthy diet?

EXERCISE 2.

Choose an elderly patient or client whom you are caring for at the moment. Observe them at meal times over a few days and answer the following questions:

Did the person usually eat everything on the plate?

If not, what did they leave?

Did they leave the same type of food each time?

If they continue to leave this type of food over a long period, what nutrients might they become deficient in?

Ask the client whether they are leaving a food because they don't like it, or because they have difficulty eating it. Looking at the eatwell plate, can you offer suggestions to the client on how to include any alternative foods of similar nutritional value?

2 Malnutrition and monitoring people who may be at risk of malnutrition

KEY POINTS

- The consequences of malnutrition can be profound.
- Many factors can affect an elderly person's eating and increase their risk of becoming malnourished.
- It can take considerable time to correct the physical and psychological effects of malnutrition in older people.
- Specific causes of malnutrition must be identified early and action taken.
- Older people are more at risk of dehydration than other groups.
- There are various methods of monitoring people who may be at risk of malnutrition.

Malnutrition is the term used to describe the clinical effects of inadequate intake of dietary energy (calories). Acute illness and disability can impact on the nutritional status of older people and the consequences of malnutrition can be profound.

People who do not take enough energy in their diet are unlikely to take in enough of the other important nutrients such as protein, vitamins and minerals. Table 2.1 describes some of the effects of malnutrition in older people.

Table 2.1 Effects of malnutrition in older people

Effect	Mechanism
Weight loss	with muscle wasting, a decrease in muscle strength, mobility and immunity
Increased risk of pressure sores	due to a loss of fat and poor mobility
Increased liability to heart failure	muscle wasting in the heart muscle
Increased risk of pneumonia and other chest infections	weakened respiratory muscles
Slower healing of wounds	may result from zinc deficiency
Altered structure of small intestine	may result in poor absorption of nutrients

The primary cause of malnutrition is a reduced intake of food. A malnourished older person is likely to have a greater risk of becoming ill, may take longer to recover and rehabilitate after illness and therefore have a longer stay in hospital. Table 2.2 shows just some of the many factors that can affect an elderly person's eating and increase their risk of becoming malnourished:

Table 2.2
Factors contributing to malnutrition

Social Factors
these mainly apply to people in their own homes

- Difficulties in shopping and/or cooking/washing up afterwards due to lack of mobility
- No appetite due to anxiety or depression
- Confusion or forgetfulness
- Living alone/feelings of social isolation or loneliness/loss of spouse
- Low budget for food/poverty

Physical Factors
these may apply to people in their own homes or in care homes

- Symptoms of illness/treatment/medicines, e.g. sickness, sore mouth, abdominal discomfort, diarrhoea
- Swallowing difficulties
- Difficulty self-feeding due to disability or diseases such as Parkinson's
- Difficulty chewing due to dental problems, dentures that don't fit or poor oral hygiene

Institutional Factors
these apply to people in hospitals and care homes

- Food unfamiliar/not to patient's liking
- Lack of storage for patient's own food
- Not enough staff to assist with feeding
- No facilities for able-bodied residents to make drinks or snacks
- Fear of asking for assistance
- Special cutlery/plates required but not provided

DEMENTIA

Patients who suffer from dementia are at risk of becoming malnourished. Dementia usually has a considerable effect on nutritional status, with malnutrition and underweight being common in sufferers. It is not a symptom of the illness itself, but a result of the impact it has on the individual's food intake. Some of the factors that may contribute to poor nutrition in dementia sufferers include:

- difficulty in shopping and cooking

- forgetting to eat
- unusual food choices and possibly gorging
- food may be held in the mouth but not swallowed
- sufferers may attempt to eat objects that are not food
- ability to use cutlery or feed self may be lost
- activity levels and hence energy expenditure may increase as a result of wandering/pacing
- patients may be reluctant to eat due to paranoia or confusion
- the patient cannot initiate movement to open the mouth or chew
- dysphagia (difficulty swallowing – see below)
- side effects of medication can include dry mouth, altered taste and sedative effect
- care staff may not have adequate time to persevere with slow eaters.

In order to maintain optimum nutritional status in patients with dementia, carers should follow the advice detailed below:

- Offer small, frequent meals and snacks.
- Fortify food wherever possible (see Chapter 3).
- Provide foods that clients can manage to eat by themselves, increasing the number of finger foods if there is difficulty using utensils.
- Offer foods the person likes regularly, whilst also trying to include variation to ensure a variety of nutrients in the diet.
- A client may eat more at certain times of the day than others; use such times as an opportunity to offer foods with high energy values such as those that have been fortified (see Chapter 3).
- Keep the table free from clutter and unnecessary objects like condiments, vases, etc. Also minimise distractions in general, such as noise from radio and television.
- Ensure the food is an appropriate texture.
- Allow sufficient time to assist patients at meal times.
- Monitor food and fluid intake (see Chapter 3).

DYSPHAGIA

Dysphagia is the term used when a person's ability to swallow is impaired. It is potentially a fatal condition if sufferers attempt to swallow foods or liquid that they are unable to swallow. This can result in passage of food into the lungs, where food 'goes down the wrong way'. This is termed 'aspiration'. If patients continue to aspirate regularly they will suffer from chest infections, or even pneumonia.

Some common causes of dysphagia are:

- stroke
- Parkinson's disease

- spinal injury/deformity
- multiple sclerosis
- stricture or spasm in oesophagus
- cerebral palsy
- cancer in neck or head area
- Huntington's disease
- injury or surgery to the mouth, lips or tongue
- motor neurone disease.

Dysphagia affects the nutritional status of sufferers in a number of ways. Eating can become slow and tiring for the patient and they may not be able to eat a sufficient amount or variety of food to meet their nutritional requirements. This will lead to weight loss and the other consequences of malnutrition detailed above. Dysphagia may have psychological effects on an individual's ability to eat, for example, fear of choking or depression due to the changes caused by their illness.

Meeting the Nutritional Needs of Dysphagic Patients

Patients with swallowing difficulties are identified during an assessment which may be performed initially by a specially trained nurse, and then more thoroughly by a speech and language therapist (SLT). The SLT will carry out oral trials with the patient, and they will be able to tell what sort of foods the patient can safely eat. The food may have to be made into a particular texture that is appropriate for their swallowing ability. This is termed texture modification, and common terms used are: soft, soft mashed, mashed, puree.

Patients may or may not be able to swallow normal fluids, so their drinks may have to be thickened to an appropriate consistency. These may be termed syrup thick, or custard thick. Thickening fluids prevents them from falling down the throat too quickly and causing choking. Thickening is achieved using commercial thickening agents, but ready thickened drinks are also available. When caring for patients with dysphagia, your employer should ensure that you have adequate training in the use of thickeners and texture modified diets. This can be delivered by somebody in your organisation who is suitably trained, or your district's SLT team.

Patients who are on texture modified diets are limited to foods that can be suitably retextured for use. The texture of foods like bread, fresh fruits, pulses and some meats can be difficult or impossible to modify. These may be excluded from the diet, and hence so are the nutrients that they contain. Patients and their carers should be guided by the eatwell plate model (see Chapter 1), and try to incorporate as many foods as possible into their diet. Hospitals and care homes may make their puree diets on the premises, or they can be bought in ready made. The same goes for patients living in their own homes; although readymade puree meals are expensive to buy. When involved in the nutritional care of dysphagic patients, the following points should be noted:

- The patient may not tolerate sufficient quantities of foods to meet daily energy and protein needs.

- Pureed food may have had extra water added to achieve the correct texture – this will have a diluting effect on the nutritional value. Consider fortifying the food (see Chapter 3).
- Dysphagic patients are at high risk of dehydration. Making sure that fluids are not only thickened to the correct consistency, but that they are at an appropriate temperature and a flavour the patient likes will encourage the patient to drink.
- Pureed food does not look very appetising when it is mixed up into an unattractive brownish mass. Try to keep the different elements of the meal separate if possible.
- Ensure the patient's posture is comfortable for eating. The back should be as straight as possible.

There may be reasons that elderly people become malnourished other than those outlined in this chapter. The important point to remember is that the specific causes of malnutrition must be identified and action taken.

IDENTIFYING PEOPLE AT RISK OF MALNUTRITION

It is important that nutritional risk is identified early. It can take considerable time to correct the physical and psychological effects of malnutrition in older people. Those who are ill are at greater risk of malnutrition as their food intake may be reduced as a consequence.

SCREENING TOOLS

Hospital or care home workers may have experience of using the MUST tool (Malnutrition Advisory Group, 2003) or a local nutrition risk screening tool. Every patient should have one of these completed on admission. Domiciliary care workers may not have seen a malnutrition screening tool before, but should acquire one and try to understand how it works. Many NHS trusts will have developed a screening tool that is suitable for use in the community – these tend to be straightforward and easy to use. They can take the form of a flowchart or checklist and there is often a scoring system for malnutrition risk. Your line manager may have a copy of the tool; if not contact your local dietitians and they will be able to provide one and possibly deliver some training on its use.

What are the warning signs that a patient may be at risk of malnutrition and what action might I take?

Table 2.3
Signs of malnutrition and actions to take

Signs	Suggested Action
Weight loss - Clothes do not fit properly - Jewellery, such as rings and watches, looks too big - Signs of weakness and reduced mobility	Weigh patient weekly if possible and if they consent to this Record weight If weighing not possible, make a record of any observations Report to care manager or staff nurse

Signs	Suggested Action
Evidence of poor food intake • Food being left on plate • Food being thrown away • Food being hidden • Food in store cupboard/fridge/freezer remains unused • No evidence of scraps in bin or used crockery	Ask the patient gently if there is a problem Discreetly suggest to the client why you have cause for concern Do not confront or embarrass the person Report to your line manager
Changes in appetite/oral health • Refusing food • Complaining of loss of appetite • Feeling or being sick • Not interested in food • Poor oral hygiene • Dentures that no longer fit comfortably	Ask why the patient is refusing Try asking them if there is anything that would tempt them Suggest patient contacts GP if feeling or being sick Suggest patient makes an appointment with their dentist Report to your line manager

NB if you work in domiciliary care and wish to record a patient's weight, you should familiarise yourself with the company's documentation policy.

WHAT ABOUT FLUIDS?

Older people are more at risk of dehydration than other groups due to the following factors:

- The thirst mechanism becomes less sensitive as we get older.
- The kidneys do not work as well as the body ages.
- The skin becomes thinner with age so more fluid is lost by this route.
- Some people may not be able to get themselves a drink.
- People who are confused or have dementia may forget to have a drink.
- People with mobility problems may be put off drinking enough due to the need to pass water more frequently.

In older people the effects of dehydration can include:

- loss of skin elasticity
- constipation
- increased risk of pressure sores

Malnutrition and monitoring people who may be at risk

- confusion
- altered heart function
- drowsiness
- increased risk of urinary infections
- electrolyte imbalances (salts).

It is important to remember that a fluid loss of 20% can be fatal in an older person. To prevent chronic dehydration, an elderly person needs about 6–8 drinks per day, each being about 150–200mls and in the correct type of cup for ease of handling. This can include hot beverages as well as water and juice. More fluid will be obtained from foods like soup.

MONITORING PEOPLE WHO MAY BE AT RISK OF MALNUTRITION

Weight/BMI

Hospital and care home workers should have access to digital weighing scales that are designed for medical use, and are calibrated regularly. It is good practice to weigh patients on admission to hospital and calculate their BMI (Body Mass Index). This should be repeated weekly for in-patients. Patients in residential care should be weighed monthly as routine, except those patients who are considered to be at nutritional risk (see below); such individuals should be weighed weekly.

In the vast majority of cases, weight is a good indicator of nutritional status. However, there are a few exceptions where weight alone cannot be relied upon, as in the following list:

- Shifts in fluid balance can cause weight loss (if the patient takes diuretic medication) or weight gain. This should be taken into consideration, particularly in oedematous or ascitic patients (patients who retain fluid in the limbs, or in the abdomen). Accurate fluid balance charts will confirm if this is the case.

- When weighing patients in plaster casts, make sure to write on the weight chart something like 'weighed with plaster cast in situ'. This is usually overlooked, and after removal it can appear that there has been considerable weight loss.

- When using digital sit-on scales, ensure that patient's feet are on both footrests, or the weight reading will be inaccurate. Also make sure that their handbag or other such personal possessions do not end up on the scales with them.

BMI is the term used for an individual's weight for height ratio. There are various charts available for calculating BMI, but it can be calculated using the formula $\frac{\text{WEIGHT (kg)}}{\text{HEIGHT}^2 \text{ (m)}}$

The healthy range is 20–25.
For example, a person who is 1.70m tall and weighs 65 kg has a BMI of 22.5, which falls in the healthy range.
A BMI of less than 18.5 is classified as underweight.
A BMI of more than 25 is classified as overweight.

Malnutrition and monitoring people who may be at risk

There is no universally accepted definition of malnutrition, but a person can be considered to be at nutritional risk if:

- they have a BMI of less than 18.5
- they have unintentionally lost more than 10% of their body weight in 3–6 months
- they are acutely ill and there has been or is likely to be no nutritional intake for more than five days.

In the appendices, you will find an example of a weight chart. Hospital and residential care workers will probably use these. Home care workers may not be using weight charts at present but may photocopy and use the one provided if they wish (with their line manager's permission). Remember always to gain the consent of the client, and follow your organisation's documentation policy.

FOOD RECORD CHART

A food record chart is a monitoring tool used to keep a record of a person's food and fluid intakes. They are useful especially where there is more than one individual involved in a client's care. Provided they are filled in correctly and with sufficient detail, they can be used as evidence when reporting to your line manager – for example, if you are worried that a client is not eating as well as they used to, or they are, or appear to be, losing weight. If a dietitian becomes involved in the client's care, food record charts will be useful for assessment and can assist them in formulating a care plan.

Those who work in hospitals and care homes will be familiar with food charts, but domiciliary workers may not have seen them before. Although these charts are usually filled in at the request of a dietitian, there is no reason why you should not start doing so yourself if you have concerns.

Chart 2.1
Example of a food record chart that is NOT filled in correctly

Day	Breakfast/ Drink	Snack/ drink	Lunch/ drink	Snack/ drink	Evening Meal/drink	Supper or snacks/drink
Monday	Porridge		Sandwich	Biscuit	Cooked dinner	Horlicks
Tuesday	Tea and toast		Soup and sandwich		Potatoes and meat	Jam sandwich
Wednesday	Toast	Milk	Soup tea		Frozen meal	Paste sandwich

Points to note:

- Use the sections as prompts, i.e. if there is a section then that information is required and should be filled in and not skipped (see examples below).
- Always state the amount of food eaten.
- Record any nutritional supplements the client has taken.
- Seven days worth of records will usually give you enough evidence to support your theory that a person may be at nutritional risk. You can use them longer term if you want to.
- Confidentiality issues should be kept in mind.
- Last but not least, **gain the client's (or carer's or relative's) consent.**

Malnutrition and monitoring people who may be at risk

Chart 2.2
Example of a food record chart that IS filled in correctly

Day	Breakfast/ Drink	Snack/ drink	Lunch/ drink	Snack/ drink	Evening Meal/drink	Supper or snacks/drink
Monday	½ bowl of porridge/ cup of tea		Cheese sandwich all eaten/ cup of tea	Biscuit/ Cup of tea	Mash, peas and chop ¾ eaten/ Small bowl ice cream all eaten/ cup of tea	Mug of horlicks all drunk
Tuesday	2 slices toast with butter and full cup of tea	½ glass of milk	None - refused soup and sandwich. Drank cup of tea		Potatoes and mince ½ plateful eaten/ cup of tea	Jam sandwich (2 slices bread) all eaten Mug of Horlicks
Wednesday	1 slice toast and butter cup of tea		½ tin of Soup/ cup of tea		Frozen fish pie All eaten	Paste sandwich (1 slice bread)/ Horlicks

Diet history

A person's diet history is a snapshot of what their typical day's food and drink intake looks like. It can be a good indicator of the person's food preferences, dislikes and what sort of times they eat. Details such as this may be seen in the personal information section of the nursing notes at your place of work. If you work alone in home care, you may visit a client not knowing much about their preferences in food. In either case, a diet history is useful in revealing whether the food that is provided for the patient/client is similar to or different from what they usually have. If a client/patient has communication difficulties, you may use picture cards or whatever aids are available on the ward, care home or for domiciliary workers in the client's home already. In the event of a person being unable to communicate verbally or using aids, then their relatives or main carer should be contacted to obtain the information.

POINT FOR REFLECTION

You may have experienced unusual circumstances that have affected an elderly person's eating. Write a brief account, or list any other factors you can think of.

EXERCISE 3

Work out your own BMI and that of a few volunteers by using a chart, or the equation.

$$\frac{\text{WEIGHT (kg)}}{\text{HEIGHT}^2 \text{ (m)}}$$

You will then feel confident to work out the BMI of your clients.

Malnutrition and monitoring people who may be at risk

EXERCISE 4

Before completing this exercise gain the permission of your line manager and the consent of the client.

See the examples in the text of food record charts that are filled in correctly and incorrectly. Practice filling in a food record chart for a client using the food record chart in the appendices at the back of the book. Keep the sheet as a master copy, and make photocopies for use at work.

EXERCISE 5

Diet history

You will find a diet history sheet in the appendices at the back of the book. Keep this as an original and make photocopies to use for the exercise, and place in client records (with the consent of your line manager).

You will find a list of example questions below that will enable you to take a detailed diet history. First, fill out a diet history sheet for yourself and perhaps a family member. Then do the same with a colleague. Once you feel happy that you have taken a thorough diet history from a colleague, try with a client.

Example questions:

Do you have breakfast? What do you have?

Do you have a snack or drink mid-morning or do you not eat again until lunch?

Do you have lunch? What sorts of foods do you tend to have? Do you have a dessert or sweet? Do you have a drink?

Do you have a snack or drink in the afternoon, or do you not eat again until your evening meal?

Do you have a meal in the evening/at tea time? What would it be usually? Do you have a dessert or sweet? Do you have a drink?

Do you have any supper, snacks or drinks during the evening? What about alcohol?

Do you use full fat, semi-skimmed or skimmed milk?

On your bread and toast, do you have low fat spread or butter?

Malnutrition and monitoring people who may be at risk

CASE STUDY

Mrs Ditchfield is a 82-year-old lady with a diagnosis of early dementia, living in a nursing and residential home. She usually eats at every meal, but recently has not been finishing her meals and has started to get up from the table and wander around the dining room. When asked why, she states that she does not like the food. You have noticed that Mrs Ditchfield seems to be losing weight. You mention this to your line manager, who asks you to monitor her and report to her at the end of the week.

EXERCISE 6

Look at the case study above.

What monitoring tools would you use for this lady to give your manager the information she requires? Give reasons why these would be appropriate.

How might you help to encourage Mrs Ditchfield to be more settled at meal times, and perhaps eat more?

3 Food Fortification and Nutritional Supplements

KEY POINTS

- Fortifying food increases its nutritional value without necessarily increasing the volume.
- Food fortification should be used as a first line treatment whenever possible.
- Nutritional supplements can be used to meet the nutritional requirements of patients for whom food fortification is not appropriate.

FOOD FORTIFICATION

This means enriching the food a person eats every day and increasing its calorie and protein value. This may be appropriate when a person feels they may like to gain weight, or if they have lost weight, to prevent this happening any further. It may be that they have a small appetite, so fortifying their food will increase its nutritional value without the client having to increase the amount of food they eat. Dietitians usually advise food fortification as a first line treatment, and it is important that this advice is followed. They usually provide instructions on how to do this. This advice will have been given after a full assessment of the patient's needs. The dietetic department of your local hospital may have leaflets containing information on food fortification that will be appropriate for your use.

General Guidelines for Food Fortification

- Add 4-6 teaspoons of dried milk powder to 1 pint of full fat milk. Shake well and refrigerate. Use the milk for drinking on its own, adding to tea, coffee or any hot beverage, on cereals/porridge, adding to mashed potato/puddings, to make up Horlicks, Ovaltine, hot chocolate.
- Add dried milk powder to soups, stews, rice puddings etc., but not too much as it will alter the taste or texture of the food.
- Add double cream or evaporated milk to any suitable foods such as desserts and tinned fruit.
- Add cheese to foods such as mashed potato, top of shepherds pie and omelettes.
- Use butter or margarine on sandwiches, toast, mashed potatoes etc., rather than low fat spread.
- Add extra sugar, honey or jam to sweet foods unless the patient is diabetic.
- Use full fat versions of dairy foods like yoghurt and cheese spread.

Food fortification and nutritional supplements

NB *Before assisting a client to begin any dietary changes that may involve increasing intakes of saturated fat or hydrogenated fat, make sure they have checked with their GP that this is ok. Some people with high blood fat levels, who have diabetes or who are on certain medication may be advised NOT to increase their fat intake.*

NUTRITIONAL SUPPLEMENTS

These are products that are prescribed by a health professional when a patient is not meeting their nutritional requirements with diet alone. They may have a poor appetite, especially during illness and be unable to consume enough food to provide the body with sufficient energy and protein. Nutritional supplements should be prescribed after a thorough nutritional assessment has been performed by a suitably qualified person.

Many of the nutritional supplements that are being used by patients are regarded as drugs for the management of certain conditions, particularly disease-related malnutrition. As such, they should be prescribed by a health professional, who will ensure that the patient is adequately monitored. The products are available in a variety of forms: ready-to-drink sip feeds, shakes, soups, powders and liquids that are used to fortify food, semi-solid (custard consistency and served in a tub), and should always be taken as directed. In the sections below the nutritional supplements are described and the names of some examples are given.

Sip feeds

These are usually presented ready to drink in cartons or bottles. They can be milkshake style or juice style and are available in a variety of flavours. They normally contain micronutrients (vitamins and minerals) as well as carbohydrate and protein. Some may also contain added fibre. Sip feeds are more palatable if they are served cold straight from the fridge. Below is a list of some sip feeds that are commonly used both on hospital wards and for people living in their own homes:

- Clinutren
- Ensure Plus
- Enlive Plus
- Enrich
- Fortijuice
- Fortisip
- Fresubin Energy
- Provide Extra
- Resource

Please note that sip feed supplements that are opened and kept at room temperature must be thrown away after 4 hours. Supplements that are opened and kept in the fridge should be thrown away after 24 hours.

Food fortification and nutritional supplements

Shakes

Shakes are powders usually presented in sachets within a box. They are normally added to milk to make a milk shake. They do not usually contain vitamins and minerals but are good sources of energy and protein. When mixed with whole (full cream) milk, the energy value will be higher than if made up with semi-skimmed or skimmed milk. Like sip feeds, these should be served cold. See examples below:

- Calshake
- Complan Shake
- Scandishake

Semi-solids

Semi-solids can be eaten with a spoon from the carton in which they are presented. They are the consistency of thick custard and taste sweet like a milk-based pudding. They come in a variety of flavours and are particularly useful when a liquid supplement would not be appropriate, for example in a dysphagic patient who is on a texture modified diet. Here are some example products:

- Clinutren Dessert
- Forticreme Complete
- Resource Dessert

Powders and liquids added to food to fortify it

Food fortification can be carried out without prescription using everyday foodstuffs. However, some patients may be prescribed specific food fortification supplements. These can be in the form of a powder or liquid, which is mixed into the patient's food and drinks. They should be tasteless and odourless so as not to deter the patient from eating the food. For example:

- Calogen*
- Caloreen
- Duocal
- Maxijul
- Pro-Cal
- Pro-Cal Shot*
- Polycal
- Polycose
- Quickcal
- Vitajoule

*Please note these two liquid products are often given in 30ml doses as an oral medicine rather than mixed in food.

Soups

These are usually instant soups made up with boiling water. For example:

- Vegenat – med
- Vitasavoury

If nutritional supplements are prescribed, they should be given as directed, and included on food record charts if these are in use. Please note that it is unlikely that you will be able to thicken sip feeds or shakes to modified consistencies.

POINT FOR REFLECTION

Patients do not always take nutritional supplements that have been prescribed for them. Think about why this may happen and write down a few points.

EXERCISE 7

Following on from the point for reflection above, it will help you to understand the viewpoint of patients who are on supplements if you try them yourself. Ask your line manager if you may take some nutritional supplements home in order to complete this exercise. Put some supplements in the fridge for several hours or overnight, and leave the others in a warm room. Taste both the chilled and the un-chilled drinks and write a brief account of your thoughts.

If possible, it would be worthwhile trying to perform this tasting exercise in your place of work along with a few colleagues. In many hospital wards, and some care homes, sip feeds are kept at room temperature on medicine trolleys or in treatment rooms. Experiencing the impact temperature can have on the palatability of nutritional supplements may motivate staff to keep these refrigerated, whilst enhancing patient compliance and reducing waste.

Food fortification and nutritional supplements

> **CASE STUDY**
>
> Mr Dobbs is a 74-year-old gentleman who lives in his own home. After a recent fall, he has returned home from a rehabilitation ward with a care package. He has two visits per day – in the morning the carer prepares his breakfast and a sandwich for his lunch, which she leaves in the fridge. At 4.30 she prepares his evening meal.
>
> Mr Dobbs has been complaining that since his fall, he has lost weight and would like to 'put a bit back on'. He says his appetite is not as good as it was since he does not exercise as much as he used to, so he cannot eat any more than his three average size meals a day. Mr Dobbs has a BMI within the normal range – at 1.76m tall he weighs 67kg. However, he had been 72kg prior to his fall.

EXERCISE 8

Look at the case study above.

What would you suggest to help Mr Dobbs gain some weight?

4 Special Dietary Needs

KEY POINTS

- Elderly people have the widest range of chronic diseases of any client group.
- They may find dietary changes quite challenging if it means avoiding food that they have enjoyed all their lives.
- A decline in the senses of taste and smell due to ageing can discourage patients from following advice.

DIABETES

There are two types of diabetes: type 1 where patients are always treated with diet and insulin, and type 2 where they are treated with diet alone, diet and tablets or diet and insulin. In type 1 diabetes, little or no insulin is produced by the patient's body. In type 2, there is some insulin production but the body cannot use it effectively. Diabetes cannot be cured, but can be managed well if patients are compliant with medication, dietary advice and screening. There are complications associated with diabetes (see list below), but effective management can slow the progression of the condition and sufferers may not necessarily develop all of these:

- Retinopathy – this affects the blood vessels in the eye and can lead to blindness.
- Nephropathy – this affects the kidneys and can cause kidney failure.
- Neuropathy – this affects the extremities of the body and is characterised by loss of sensation, poor circulation and can lead to infection. Gangrene may occur and ultimately limb amputation.
- Cardiovascular disease – poor control of diabetes leads to higher blood fat levels, high blood pressure and sufferers are at risk of stroke.

Blood glucose should ideally be 4–7 mmol/litre before a meal. Diabetic patients who are capable of doing so will be taught by a diabetes nurse to test their own blood samples at appropriate intervals. The aim of diabetes treatment is to alleviate the symptoms of the disease and reduce the risk of diabetes complications. Diet is an integral part of treatment and it is recommended that patients follow the same healthy eating guidelines as the healthy adult population (see Chapter 1) with a few adaptations. This means:

- carbohydrate foods should form the largest part of meals and snacks. People with diabetes should be encouraged to eat lower GI versions of regular foods, such as wholemeal bread, wholegrain or oat based cereals;
- at least five fruit and vegetables per day should be eaten;
- milk and dairy foods should be eaten every day. Lower fat versions of

Special dietary needs

these should be eaten due to the risk of cardiovascular complications in diabetes. Yogurts which are low fat can sometimes be high in sugar. Diabetic patients should aim for those which contain less than 10g of sugar per 100g;

- some meat, fish, eggs, beans and other non-dairy sources of protein should be eaten every day. It is recommended that two portions of fish per week should be eaten, one of which should be oily. It is important that fat should be removed from meat and skin from poultry, and that methods of cooking that reduce fat intake are used, such as grilling rather than frying. High fat meat products such as burgers, pies and sausage rolls should be eaten only occasionally. Patients should be encouraged to eat more pulses;

- high fat/high sugar foods should generally be avoided, in favour of low fat/low sugar alternatives, for example, diet or no added sugar versions of soft drinks and jams;

- plain biscuits such as digestives or rich tea may be eaten as a snack but no more than two.

Table 4.1 can be used for guidance when reading food labels to assist your patients in making healthier choices.

Table 4.1
Reading food labels

	Low	High
Sugars per 100g	Less than 2g	More than 10g
Fat per 100g	Less than 3g	More than 20g
Saturated fat per 100g	Less than 1g	More than 5g
Fibre per 100g	Less than 0.5g	More than 3g
Sodium per 100g	Less than 0.1g	More than 0.5g

NAGE (Nutrition Advisory Group for Elderly People) have produced an excellent leaflet titled *Eating Well and Keeping Well with Diabetes*; see recommended reading list.

HYPOGLYCAEMIA

Patients who are on medication especially insulin are at risk of hypoglycaemia (low blood sugar), or 'hypos'. Symptoms of this are: sweating, shaking, increased heart rate, confusion, disorientation, slurred speech and aggression. The behaviour can often be mistaken for drunkenness. Hypos can be caused by missing a meal, not eating enough carbohydrates, alcohol consumption (especially if on an empty stomach). To avoid hypos, it is important that patients:

- have regular meals

- eat plenty of starchy carbohydrate foods (see Chapter 1) at each meal – these should make up one-third of the meal

- should not miss a meal

- should always carry an emergency supply of carbohydrate, for example, glucose tablets or drink

Special dietary needs

- should not exceed the safe drinking limit of 3–4 units per day for men and 2–3 units for women. However, it is recommended that people with diabetes should have at least three alcohol-free days per week. Patients on insulin should consume some food containing carbohydrate before and after consuming alcohol as alcohol has a hypoglycaemic effect, i.e. it lowers blood sugar.

If a patient becomes hypoglycaemic, their confused state may cause them to forget what they are supposed to do to treat themselves. You should encourage and assist them to consume their emergency carbohydrates. Once they have recovered, they should be offered a snack of slower acting carbohydrates such as a sandwich or milk and biscuits to prevent this from happening again. If the patient becomes unconscious they will need a glucagon injection to bring them round, and some carbohydrate soon after. Families and carers of patients who are at risk of severe hypos should be trained to use these. Otherwise, emergency medical assistance should be summoned as coma and death can occur if a hypo is not treated.

COELIAC DISEASE

Coeliac disease is a condition that results from an intolerance to gluten, a protein found in wheat and rye. Similar proteins found in barley and oats can trigger the same reaction in some people. The consumption of these proteins in the diet leads to damage to cells in the intestines. This impacts on the general health of the patients as they cannot absorb vital nutrients from their food effectively. The condition is permanent, and the sufferer must exclude gluten from their diet on a permanent basis in order to correct the damage to the intestine and reduce the risk of nutritional deficiency. Wheat ingredients are used in many foods, most types of bread, pasta, pizza, pastry and cakes, as a filler in foods like sausages and burgers, and many sauces. Foods in batter or breadcrumbs are unsuitable for people with coeliac disease, as are beer and lager. To comply with food labelling rules in the UK and the EU, it must be stated clearly on the label if a food (or any of its ingredients) contains cereals containing gluten, including wheat, rye, barley and oats. It is important that patients replace staple foods such as bread with other forms of carbohydrate to ensure that they take enough energy in their diet. When a patient is diagnosed with coeliac disease, they will be given advice from a dietitian on which foods are suitable and which should be avoided.

Elderly patients with coeliac disease may find the condition particularly challenging, especially if it means changing habits that have developed over a lifetime. They may be confused, or need help to make appropriate food choices, especially in reading food labels. They will need to avoid ordinary bread and pastry, which are foods they are familiar with, and may struggle to come to terms with having to eat things which are unfamiliar. They can have specially made gluten-free bread, crackers, pasta and flour which is available on prescription. If they are relying on carers, staff should familiarise themselves with foods that are suitable. Some processed foods such as sauces, gravy, desserts and crisps contain gluten as an additive. Food that is prepared for coeliac patients should not come into contact with food that contains gluten, as cross-contamination will occur and the patient can unintentionally ingest gluten in this way. Cross-contamination can occur in many ways:

- Gluten-free bread may be placed on surfaces such as boards that have been used to cut or butter ordinary bread.
- There may be remnants of bread or toast crumbs that find their way into butter, margarine or jam from knives that have been used on ordinary bread by non-coeliac family members.
- Toasters and grill pans can harbour bread crumbs.
- Deep fat fryers can contain wheat remnants from foods such as fish or chicken covered in batter or breadcrumbs.

Coeliac UK provides a wide range of written materials to support patients and their carers, including a directory of gluten-free foods. When caring for coeliac patients, you should make sure you obtain a directory, or that the patient's own copy is always available for your reference, and that it is up to date. Some foods are naturally gluten-free and if they have not undergone any processing are safe to eat. For example:

- Cornflakes
- Rice cereals
- Fresh/frozen/tinned/dried fruit
- Fresh/frozen/tinned vegetables
- Peas/lentils/beans (check label if canned)
- Nuts
- Milk
- Cheese
- Cream
- Most yogurts
- Meat
- Chicken
- Fish (not battered)
- Jam
- Tea
- Coffee
- Juice
- Wine

This is a very short list, and the directory should be consulted for detailed information. An older person with coeliac disease should follow the same healthy eating guidelines as the healthy older person, and include a variety of foods from all the food groups. For the coeliac patient, this may mean having meals that are made from unprocessed ingredients such as potatoes, meat or fish and vegetables. This can be more time-consuming and involve more physical effort than using convenience foods. Carers looking after patients in their own homes should be aware that assisting in meal preparation may require a longer than average call. Staff in hospitals and care homes should ensure that food brought in by visitors is suitable, especially if the patient is forgetful and may not realise that what they are eating is inappropriate.

LOW SALT DIETS

The Food Standards Agency has set a target for the adult population to reduce the average salt consumption to 6g a day by 2010; healthy older adults are obviously included in this group. Consuming too much salt can increase the risk of hypertension (high blood pressure), heart disease and stroke. Most of the salt eaten by the general public is taken in processed foods. During processing and preservation salt or additives that contain it are added to prolong shelf life and stability. Many people also add salt at the table and in cooking. Unprocessed foods in their natural state contain only small mounts of naturally occurring sodium. Salt is made up of two components – sodium and chloride. You may see salt content expressed as sodium on food labels. To convert to salt content, multiply this figure by 2.5.

Patients can require a diet that is low in salt for a variety of reasons, such as kidney, heart or liver disease. The average person's diet would need to contain fewer packaged and processed foods, and more fresh unprocessed foods to make a significant impact on sodium intake. More severe restrictions on sodium are necessary in patients with certain diseases. These restrictions are classified as no added salt and low salt, as described below.

No added salt: 80–100mmol sodium per day

- Patients should use only a pinch of salt in cooking, and should not add salt at the table or to cooked food.

- Herbs and spices can be used to flavour food, except those which contain salt such as garlic salt.

- The following foods should be avoided: tinned meat, bacon, cured meats, ham, sausages, meat pastes or pates, pies, pasties, sausages, smoked fish, tinned fish in brine or tomato sauce, savoury biscuits, tinned vegetables in salt water, tinned and packet soups, Oxo, Marmite, Bovril, stock cubes, gravy powder/granules, soya sauce, bottled sauce/chutney and salted or flavoured nuts and crisps. All these contain high levels of added salt.

- Use the alternative foods listed below instead: fresh and frozen meat, fresh unsmoked fish, tinned fish in oil or water, milk, eggs, cream, yoghurt, cottage cheese, bread, biscuits, rice, pasta, fats and oils, all fruits, all fresh or frozen vegetables, tea, coffee, squash, fizzy drinks, fruit juice, home made soups without salt, unsalted nuts, salt and shake crisps, but without adding the salt in the sachet.

- Avoid the following food additives which are high in sodium: monosodium glutamate, sodium nitrite and sodium bicarbonate.

- Limit hard cheese to 125 g (4 oz) per week.

- Limit bread to 4 slices per day.

Low salt: 40mmol sodium per day

The advice above should be followed, but in addition the following restrictions apply:

- No salt may be used in cooking or at the table.
- Salt free margarine or butter must be used.
- Breakfast cereals must be low in salt, e.g. shredded wheat or puffed wheat.
- Milk should be limited to 300ml per day.

There have been many studies that show that older people have low compliance with low salt diets. Older people living in their own homes may find salt restriction particularly challenging, especially with regard to purchasing, storing and preparing unprocessed foods. Such foods can be perishable in a short period of time, and may be perceived as expensive. Also, low salt diets can be bland, and a decline in the senses of taste and smell due to ageing can further discourage patients from following advice. Patients on low salt diets will have been given written materials by a dietitian, and this guidance should ideally be followed. For a home care worker, meal-time visits may require more time than usual, as with other elderly patients with special dietary needs.

LIPID-LOWERING DIET

This may also be known as a cholesterol-lowering diet, and is low in saturated and animal fats. The body requires essential fatty acids to function correctly, and these are obtained from foods containing fats. Patients who suffer from coronary heart disease are advised to follow a low fat diet. It is preferable for such patients to obtain essential fats from polyunsaturated or monounsaturated sources (sometimes known as 'good' fats) rather than saturated or trans fats. Saturated and trans fats raise the levels of a particular type of cholesterol (LDL cholesterol) in the blood which increases the risk of heart disease. Trans fats are formed when vegetable oils are turned into solid fats through the process of hydrogenation. Patients who are on lipid-lowering diets are advised to follow a healthy balanced diet as are healthy older people, with the majority of their dietary intake consisting of carbohydrates, and plenty of fruit and vegetables. Saturated and trans fats (as well as high levels of salt) can be found in the following foods, which should be avoided:

- meat products, meat pies, sausages
- hard cheeses
- butter and lard
- pastry
- cakes and biscuits
- coconut oil and palm oil
- cream, soured cream and crème fraîche
- fast food
- some margarines.

Some unsaturated fats not only provide a healthier alternative to those above, but some also help to lower cholesterol. The foods in the list below are high in unsaturated fats:

- oily fish
- avocados
- nuts and seeds
- vegetable oils
- sunflower, rapeseed and olive oil and spreads made from these.

You can assist your patients/clients in making lower fat choices by bringing their attention to the information on packaged foods.

Foods that are **high in fat** contain more than 20g fat per 100g.

Foods that are **low in fat** contain less than 3g fat per 100g.

Foods that are **high in saturated fat** contain more than 5g saturates per 100g.

Foods that are **low in saturated fat** contain less than 1.5g saturates per 100g.

As well as avoiding foods high in fat, you should observe the following advice when preparing food for patients who are on a low fat diet:

- Choose lean cuts of meat and trim off any visible fat.
- Grill, bake, poach, steam or dry roast food rather than frying.
- Domiciliary care workers who shop for their clients should (with the client's permission) when choosing ready meals or packaged foods, compare the labels and pick those with less total fat or less saturated fat.
- When you are making sandwiches for patients on a low fat diet, try not using any butter or spread if the filling is moist enough.
- Encourage patients to use reduced-fat spread or olive oil spread.
- Encourage patients to choose lower fat versions of dairy foods whenever possible. This means semi-skimmed or skimmed milk and reduced fat yoghurt.
- Encourage patients to eat plenty of soluble fibre as this may help to reduce the amount of cholesterol in the blood. Good sources of soluble fibre include oats, beans, peas, lentils, chickpeas, fruit and vegetables.

FOOD ALLERGY AND INTOLERANCE

There are eight main foods that cause allergy in the British population: milk, eggs, peanuts (groundnuts or monkey nuts), nuts (including Brazil nuts, hazelnuts, almonds and walnuts), fish, shellfish (including mussels, crab and
shrimps), soya and wheat. Wheat allergy has been covered in the earlier section on coeliac disease. A food allergy can be life-threatening, and may be triggered by minute amounts of the allergen. An allergic reaction is mediated by the immune system. The symptoms are swelling of the throat and mouth, streaming eyes and nose and difficulty in breathing. If untreated anaphylaxis can occur, which can be fatal. However, not all food

Special dietary needs

allergies cause such an extreme reaction and sometimes they appear several hours after ingestion as a skin rash. Food intolerance is a term used for reactions to food that do not involve the immune system, such as symptoms caused by a lack of an enzyme required to digest the food. These are non-life-threatening and do not cause anaphylactic shock. If you are looking after a patient with a severe food allergy, they should have a pre-loaded syringe containing adrenaline with them at all times, and their relatives and carers should be instructed how to administer the dose.

Milk allergy

Cows' milk allergy is caused by a reaction to proteins in cows' milk and people can react to whole milk, casein or whey. People with milk allergy should avoid the following foods, and should avoid any processed foods if they see any of these on the label:

- milk
- milk solids
- skimmed milk powder
- cream
- butter
- cheese
- yogurt
- whey
- lactose
- casein
- caseinates
- hydrolysed casein
- margarine
- non-fat milk solids
- ghee
- hydrolysed whey protein.

People with milk allergy should replace milk with other foods containing calcium and vitamin D. They can use the following foods as replacements, but these should have added calcium:

- soya milk
- rice milk
- oat milk
- soya cheese
- soya yogurt
- soya ice cream

Other foods that are rich sources of calcium and should be included in the diet regularly are:

- fortified breakfast cereals
- canned fish with bones
- tofu
- nuts and seeds
- bread
- dried figs
- spinach
- watercress.

Peanut allergy

Peanuts are also known as groundnuts and monkey nuts and are one of the most common causes of food allergy. It causes a severe reaction, and minute amounts of peanut can cause a reaction in people who are sensitive. Sufferers should avoid possible cross-contamination of their food, with food that contains peanuts. Even being close to someone else eating peanuts can be enough to make some people react. If a food contains peanuts or any of its ingredients contains them, then it must be declared on the food label in the UK and the EU. Some people with peanut allergy might also react to legumes such as soya, green beans, kidney beans and peas because these foods contain similar allergens to peanuts.

Shellfish allergy

Allergy to shellfish is quite common and people who are sensitive can react to one or more types of shellfish, such as shrimps, prawns, lobsters, crabs, crayfish, oysters, scallops, mussels and clams. Shellfish allergy can often cause severe reactions, and some people can react to the vapours from cooking shellfish. Pre-packed food, sold in the UK and the European Union, must show clearly on the label if it contains crustaceans (one group of shellfish) including lobster, crab, prawns and langoustines. However, other shellfish, such as mussels, scallops, oysters, whelks and squid do not need to be labelled individually.

Egg allergy

In a few cases, egg allergy can cause anaphylaxis. Egg allergy is generally more common in children than adults. Patients with an allergy to eggs should avoid foods that contain them, such as quiche, some cakes, egg noodles and pasta. Pastry products have often been glazed with egg. If a food or any of its ingredients contains egg, then it should be stated clearly on the label. The main causes of egg allergy are proteins in the white. Cooking can destroy some but not all of these proteins which means that some people might react to raw eggs but not to cooked eggs. Occasionally people with an egg allergy may react to chicken meat, and vice versa.

Soya allergy

Soya allergy is rare in adults and rarely causes anaphylaxis. As a food additive, soya flour is often used to improve the colour of pastry and bakery goods. Textured soya protein is used in processed meat products as a filler and texture improver, but is also widely used as a meat substitute in vegetarian foods. If used in processed foods, the presence of soya must be shown clearly on the label.

POINT FOR REFLECTION

What factors do you think may affect an older person's ability to comply with changing their diet in later life? List as many points as you can think of, taking into consideration social, economic and physical factors.

EXERCISE 9

Follow a low salt diet for one day – you may want to choose a day when you are not working, to minimise disruption.

Reflect on how it felt and make some notes.

1) What was the hardest part of the day?

2) What food was hardest to resist?

3) How much longer did you take to prepare your food?

4) Did you enjoy your food?

5) Did you manage to make your food flavoursome despite not using salt?

Special dietary needs

CASE STUDY

Mrs Duffy is a 78-year-old lady who has recently been diagnosed with type 2 diabetes. She is not taking any medication for this and is expected to maintain control over her blood sugar levels with diet alone. The nurse at her GP practice gave her some diabetes education, but Mrs Duffy explains to you that she did not really understand fully, and the nurse was 'talking too fast'. She knows she is 'fine with porridge or a bit of soup' and has been having either of these at each meal time but little else. Mrs Duffy has a slim build, and a BMI of 20.

EXERCISE 10

Look at the case study above.

1) Explain why Mrs Duffy may be at risk of malnutrition if she continues to exist on soup and porridge.

2) How would you help Mrs Duffy to plan a day's meals that will be suitable for her? Look back at the eatwell plate and the section on diabetes.

5 Ethnicity, Religion and Culture

KEY POINTS

- Elderly clients may be at risk of becoming malnourished if they are not provided with food that is permitted by their culture or belief system as they may refuse to eat.

- Their first language may not be English, and they may need reassurance from their visitors, relatives or an interpreter that the food is suitable.

- The principles of the eatwell plate can be applied to individuals from a range of cultural backgrounds, as their eating patterns will include carbohydrate and protein sources as well as fruit and vegetables.

Most carers will at some point experience working with clients from different ethnic and cultural backgrounds. When this happens, you should familiarise yourself with their customs and practices, especially in relation to diet. You will find in Table 5.1 details of some of the religions practiced by ethnic groups in the UK, and dietary restrictions that apply.

This provides an overview but you should source material that provides more detailed information, ask the client and their family for information or contact your local dietetic or health promotion department who may be able to assist you. It is not only food restrictions you should be familiar with, but also customs like fasting, where a person chooses to abstain from eating and/or drinking for a given period of time, in accordance with their faith. Some religions involve celebrations and feast days – there may be certain foods that are eaten only at these times.

Table 5.1 Religious food restrictions

Religion	Food Restriction
Hindu	Rarely eat beef Many Hindus are vegetarian Animal fats such as lard are not acceptable
Muslim	Any food derived from the pig, shellfish or any fish without fins or scales will not be eaten Muslims will not eat meat unless it is Halal (has been killed in a special way) Alcohol is not permitted (including in cooking and medicine)
Sikh	Do not eat beef. Many are vegetarian
Jewish	Any food derived from the pig and seafood will not be eaten Only meat that is slaughtered by the Jewish method will be eaten (the Jewish method is called Kosher) Meat and milk must not be served in the same meal and different cutlery, plates and cooking utensils are used for meat and milk

Ethnicity, religion and culture

Rastafarian   Many are vegetarian or vegan, will not eat pork, fish without fins or scales, vine fruit, preserved or processed food
May also avoid stimulants like tea, coffee and alcohol

VEGETARIAN/VEGAN

There are various reasons why an individual may follow a vegetarian diet. It may be for religious reasons, be based on their beliefs about food and health, or it may be that they are concerned about animal welfare. People may describe themselves as vegetarian if they impose the following restrictions on their diet:

- Exclude all meat, poultry, fish and products derived from animals such as rennet and gelatine; will eat milk, cheese, eggs but may insist on free range.
- May eat fish whilst avoiding any meat or poultry.

Vegetarian diets tend to be lower in saturated fat, and higher in starchy carbohydrates, fibre, fruit and vegetables than the diets of meat eaters (Hoffman *et al.* 1999). They can also be nutritionally adequate, providing a variety of foods is consumed. Vegetarians should follow the same healthy eating advice as the rest of the adult population, whilst ensuring that they eat a variety of meat substitutes, wholegrains and pulses.

VEGANISM

Vegans exclude meats, poultry, fish, eggs, dairy products and any ingredients derived from animal sources. Some may even avoid wearing materials that have been derived from animals such as leather. Vegan diets may be low in some nutrients and examples of foods that contain these can be found in Table 5.2.

Table 5.2 Sources of nutrients for Vegan diet

Nutrient	Sources appropriate for vegan diets
Iron	Fortified breakfast cereals, seaweed, dried fruit, soya flour, pulses, watercress, spinach, wheatgerm, bread, molasses
Calcium	Fortified soya milk, soya cheese, tofu, nuts and seeds, bread, dried figs, spinach, watercress
Zinc	Fortified breakfast cereals, seaweed, soya flour, pulses, watercress, wheatgerm, bread, brown rice, pumpkin seeds, sunflower seeds, nuts
Vitamin B12	Fortified breakfast cereals, other fortified products such as soya milk, meat substitutes, vegetable stock, yeast extract and vitamin supplements
Vitamin D	Exposure to sunlight, other fortified products such as soya milk, vegan margarine, soya cheese, soya yogurt, vitamin supplements
Riboflavin	Wheatgerm, yeast extract, fortified breakfast cereals, almonds, soya beans, tempeh, fortified soya milk, mushrooms, dried apricots and prunes

6 Relevant Policy Guidelines and Standards

> **KEY POINTS**
>
> - Food and nutrition are acknowledged as key areas in the National Minimum Standards – Care Homes for Older People and also the government's Dignity in Care Campaign.
> - Meal times have an impact on the quality of life of older people both in residential care and in their own homes.
> - Malnutrition costs the UK an estimated £7.3 billion a year, and over half this amount is spent on people aged 65 and over (BAPEN 2006).

NATIONAL MINIMUM STANDARDS – CARE HOMES FOR OLDER PEOPLE

Care homes in England must register with the Commission for Social Care Inspection and are required by law to ensure they are run in accordance with the Care Homes Regulations 2001. In addition to the regulations, the National Minimum Standards – Care Homes for Older People have been published by the Department of Health. These standards identify what a care provider needs to do in order to meet their legal obligations.

According to the Standards, Nutritional Screening should be undertaken on admission, periodically thereafter, and a record maintained of nutrition, including weight gain or loss, and appropriate action taken. Standard 12 states that service users should have the opportunity to exercise their choice in relation to, amongst other things, food, meals and meal times. Another area where food service is highlighted is in Standard 15. The registered person should ensure that:

- service users receive a varied, appealing, wholesome and nutritious diet, which is suited to individual assessed and recorded requirements, and that meals are taken in a congenial setting and at flexible times;
- each service user is offered three full meals each day (at least one of which must be cooked) at intervals of not more than five hours;
- hot and cold drinks and snacks are available at all times and offered regularly;
- a snack should be offered in the evening and the interval between this and breakfast the following morning should be no more than 12 hours;
- food, including liquidised/puree meals, is presented in a manner which is attractive and appealing in terms of texture, flavour, and appearance, in order to maintain appetite and nutrition;
- special therapeutic diets/feeds are provided when advised by health care and dietetic staff, including adequate provision of calcium and vitamin D;

Relevant policy guidelines and standards

- religious or cultural dietary needs are catered for as agreed at admission and recorded in the care plan and food for special occasions is available;
- there is a menu (changed regularly), offering a choice of meals in written or other formats to suit the capacities of all service users, which is given, read or explained to service users;
- meal times are unhurried with service users being given enough time to eat;
- staff are ready to offer assistance in eating where necessary, discreetly, sensitively and individually, while independent eating is encouraged for as long as possible.

DOMICILIARY CARE NATIONAL MINIMUM STANDARDS REGULATIONS

The purpose of these minimum standards is to ensure the quality of personal care and support that people receive whilst living in their own home. The standard of service an agency provides must not fall below the minimum set out in these standards. The scope of the standards is broad – they are not specific to those caring for older people, but to anybody who cares for individuals in their own home in the community. Nutritional care, in particular dietary requirements and preferences, is an area that is given a brief mention in Standard 2. For individuals who are self-funding a care needs assessment should be undertaken in the individual's own home, by a manager competent and trained for the task, covering the delivery of the services agreed. As a domiciliary care worker, if you were to start to monitor a client's nutritional status by, for example, keeping a food record chart you should read Standards 16 and 24 on record keeping.

DIGNITY IN CARE

On 14 November 2006, the Minister for Care Services, Ivan Lewis MP, launched the Dignity in Care campaign. The aim is to raise awareness around dignity in care and create a care system where there is zero tolerance of abuse and disrespect of older people. An online survey was conducted by Ivan Lewis to hear directly from the public about their own experiences of being treated with dignity in care services, or about care they had seen provided to others. The survey revealed that dignity matters to people, but that many people do not know what they should expect from a service that respects dignity. The survey was a great success with over 400 people taking part, including members of the public and professional health and social care staff.

The Dignity Challenge is a clear statement of what people can expect from a service that respects dignity. It is backed up by a series of 'dignity tests' that can be used by care providers, commissioners and service users to see how their local services are performing. The Commission for Social Care Inspection (CSCI), Social Care Institute for Excellence (SCIE) and the Care Services Improvement Partnership (CSIP) have developed an online practice guide to assist front-line workers, practitioners, managers, commissioners, as well as older people themselves and their carers to take up the Dignity Challenge. You can see this at www.scie.org.uk where detailed information can be found about what is meant by dignity in care, practical advice and tips on how you can make a difference by taking up the Dignity Challenge.

The Dignity in Care campaign is not a one-off event. It is a major priority for the Department of Health and has widespread support from stakeholders such as Age Concern, in the advocacy sector. Events and policy development around Dignity in Care will be sustained and ongoing and involve nutrition as a key area.

PROTECTED MEAL TIMES POLICY

If you work in a hospital, you may have heard of protected meal times. This means that non-urgent clinical activity is stopped, the ward is tidied, and patients are made ready for their meals. The aim of protected meal times is to provide an environment that is conducive to eating, free from unnecessary interruptions where staff can devote sufficient time to assist patients. Some hospitals operate a system whereby patients who require assistance at meal times are allocated a red tray to alert staff. In the appendices, you will see a checklist similar to the CSCI checklist that has been adapted for use on hospital wards. If your ward has a protected meal times policy in place, most or all of the boxes will be ticked. The list is not a means by which to measure your ward's performance, more a means to check that you as a carer are personally acknowledging the importance of food service to patients.

THE FOOD STANDARDS AGENCY (FSA) – FOOD SERVED TO OLDER PEOPLE IN RESIDENTIAL CARE

In 2006 the FSA issued this guidance for UK institutions. It includes advice on nutrients, food allergy and hygiene and also features example menu plans. The guidance is available to download; see further reading list (FSA 2006).

POINT FOR REFLECTION

Think of ways you can help clients to uphold their dignity at meal times, and make notes. Think particularly about those who may have difficulties feeding themselves.

EXERCISE 11

You will need to look at the checklists in the appendices to complete this exercise. If you work in a care home, look at the checklist on p. 47. If you work on a hospital ward, look at the checklist on p. 49.

Look at each item on the list, and for each write your own thoughts on the following:

Do you perform this task routinely, sometimes or never?

If never, what do you believe prevents you from doing so?

What would enable you to improve patients' experience of meal times in your work place?

Appendices

The sheets in this section can be kept as master copies.

Remember, you may be able to use any you fill in as evidence of your competencies.

Appendix 1: Diet History

Diet History

Name _____   Date _____

Weight _____   BMI _____

Breakfast	
Snack	
Lunch	
Snack	
Evening meal	
Supper/snacks/hot drinks	
Alcohol	

Appendix 2: Food Record Chart

Food Record Chart

Name _____

Week beginning (date) _____

Day	Breakfast/ Drink	Snack/ drink	Lunch/ drink	Snack/ drink	Evening Meal/drink	Supper or snacks/drink

Weight Chart

Name _____

Date	Weight

Appendix 4: Checklist for Best Practice – social care

Checklist for Best Practice
Commission for Social Care Inspection (2006)

	Y/N
Is there a full assessment of the likes and dislikes of each older person on their admission to the care home and do staff know and act upon this assessment?	
Are older people actively consulted about what food and drinks are provided and their availability in the care home?	
Do staff have the necessary skills to discover the preferences of older people with communication difficulties?	
Are older people and staff involved in the development of care plans and are these plans reviewed regularly?	
Is the number of staff available at meal times sufficient to appropriately respond to the social, physical, emotional and cultural needs of older people?	
Is there an adequate handover during shift changes to inform staff of any changes in older people's meal needs and preferences?	
Are staff adequately trained in identifying and responding to nutrition issues relating to ageing and specific health needs?	
Are staff aware of the importance of facilitating choice and promoting independence for the well-being of older people?	
Are staff aware of the importance of cultural, social and religious practices relating to meals and meal times for each person in their care?	
Do staff have an adequate understanding of nutrition and hydration issues for older people, particularly for those with common health concerns?	
Are aids and the right crockery available to support older people in retaining as much independence as possible during meal times?	
Are the tasks associated with the production, presentation and delivery of meals well co-ordinated?	
Are staff aware of their responsibilities for meeting the national minimum standards associated with the provision of high quality meals?	
Do staff have a good understanding of food hygiene standards?	

Appendix 5: Checklist for Best Practice – hospital wards

Checklist for Best Practice – hospital wards

	Y/N
Was a Nutrition Risk Score Sheet completed for the patient on admission?	
Is this reviewed regularly?	
Was a Diet History sheet filled in for the patient on admission?	
Have staff attempted to discover the preferences of older people with communication difficulties, for example, by speaking to family or care home/domiciliary care staff?	
Is the number of staff available at meal times sufficient to appropriately respond to the social, physical, emotional and cultural needs of older people?	
Is the environment prepared for meal times? Are bed tables tidied of clutter?	
Is the water jug within easy reach?	
Have you assisted patients who need it with hand washing, or have you given wet wipes to bed bound patients?	
Are used bed pans, bowls, commodes, tissues and bottles removed from bed sides, lockers and tables at meal times?	
Have patients who require it been assisted to use the toilet before meal service?	
Is there an adequate handover during shift changes to inform staff of any changes in older people's nutritional needs and preferences?	
Are staff aware of the importance of cultural, social and religious practices relating to meals and meal times for each person in their care?	
Are staff aware of the importance of facilitating choice and promoting independence for the well-being of older people?	
Are appropriate aids and crockery available to support older people to retain as much independence as possible during meal times?	

FURTHER READING

Commission for Social Care Inspection (2006). *Highlight of the Day? – Improving Meals for Older People in Care Homes*. Available online at: www.csci.org.uk/PDF/highlight_of_day.pdf

Department of Health (2006). *Dignity in Care Public Survey.* Available at: www.dh.gov.uk/PolicyAndGuidance/HealthAndSocialCareTopics/SocialCare/DignityInCare

Food Standards Agency. *Eat well, be well. Helping you make healthier choices*. Available at: www.eatwell.gov.uk/agesandstages/olderpeople/

Food Standards Agency (2006). *Food Served to Older People in Residential Care*. Available at: www.food.gov.uk/healthiereating/nutritioncommunity/care

Food Standards Agency (2007). *8 Tips for Eating Well.* Available at: www.eatwell.gov.uk/healthydiet/eighttipssection/8tips

NAGE (Nutrition Advisory Group for Elderly People) (2005). *Eating Well and Keeping Well with Diabetes*. Birmingham: British Dietetic Association.

NAGE (Nutrition Advisory Group for Elderly People) (2004). *Have You got a Small Appetite?* Birmingham: British Dietetic Association.

REFERENCES

Association of Community Health Councils of England and Wales (1997). *Hungry in Hospital?* London: ACHCEW.

BAPEN (2006). *The cost of disease-related malnutrition in the UK and economic considerations for the use of oral nutritional supplements (ONS) in adults.*
Available online at www.bapen.org.uk/pdfs/health_econ_exec_sum.pdf

Commission for Social Care Inspection (2006). *Highlight of the Day? – Improving Meals for Older People in Care Homes.*
Available online at: www.csci.org.uk/PDF/highlight_of_day.pdf

Department of Health (2001). *Care Homes for Older People National Minimum Standards.* Available at:
www.dh.gov.uk/en/Policyandguidance/SocialCare/Standardsandregulation/DH_079561

Department of Health (2003). *Domiciliary Care National Minimum Standards Regulations.* Available at:
www.dh.gov.uk/en/Policyandguidance/SocialCare/Standardsandregulation/DH_079561

Department of Health (2006). *Dignity in Care Public Survey.* Available at: www.dh.gov.uk/PolicyAndGuidance/HealthAndSocialCareTopics/SocialCare/DignityInCare

Food Standards Agency (2007). *The eatwell plate.*
Available at: www.food.gov.uk

Hoffman, I., Groenweld, M.J. & Leitzman, C. (1999). 'Nutrient intake and nutritional status of vegetarians and low meat eaters consuming a diet meeting preventive recommendations' in *American Journal of Clinical Nutrition* **70**: 626–629.

Malnutrition Advisory Group (2003). *Malnutrition Universal Screening Tool.*
Available at: www.bapen.org.uk/must_tool.html

Office for National Statistics (ONS) (2006). *National Statistics Online.*
Available at: www.statistics.gov.uk